I0707269

Gary Fradin

Gary's Guide to Weight Loss

How One Man Lost 40 Pounds and
Plans to Keep It Off

Gary Fradin

Nothing in this book should be interpreted as medical advice.

Diets all work.

Then they generally fail.

Gary Fradin

Table of Contents

Nothing in this book is intended to be, or should be construed as, medical advice. This is merely one person's account of his own weight loss and ideas about how people might follow a similar program should they wish. This book makes no claims about weight loss results or the benefits of this program to any person or group.

You should always consult a trained, licensed medical professional about any medical issues or with any medical questions. The author has no appropriate training or licenses.

Gary Fradin

Foreword

Gary asked me to write a forward to his book while we were kayaking together. I told him I would be honored to do so.

I have worked for 30 years as a primary care physician in a mixed urban / suburban environment. Over these years obesity rates have skyrocketed. I have seen it in my own practice: young and old patients, blue and white collar, it doesn't matter.

Far too many of my patients are heavier these days causing other health conditions to become more prevalent including diabetes, hypertension and heart disease.

I have had countless people come to me complaining of their inability to lose weight. The complaints are the same and the accounts of their food intake and exercise eerily similar. "I hardly eat anything" or "I eat the same amount I always have." Lacking hard data, I wonder about this.

When I ask about their activity level, they usually respond "I try to walk." They typically want to have their thyroid checked, assuming that there is a medical explanation for their weight gain and fatigue.

My message to them is always the same: "you need to cut back on your calories and become more active". Unfortunately, we never have enough time together for me to understand their lifestyles, dietary norms and physical activity habits in enough detail.

Invariably they return frustrated and unsuccessful.

Fewer than 1/10 patients actually make the changes necessary to lose weight and keep it off.

Patients such is Gary Fradin are few and far between but a joy to work with. Gary is the rare patient who understands nutrition and exercise and actively takes control of his own health.

He formulated a plan to cut his calories and increase his activity level and enjoyed spectacular results, losing over 40 pounds and getting himself into good physical shape as well.

Gary summarized the process in this readable and informative book. His recommendations are science based, useful and appropriate. I heartily recommend it.

In fact, I plan to give this book to my own patients.

Enjoy it and good luck!

Dr. David Mudd
Easton, Massachusetts
May 2021

Preface

After Covid struck, after our lives turned upside down, after my business revenues fell by 50%, after all normal routines disappeared, my doctor told me to lose weight.

I told him I was fit and healthy.

He repeated his order.

How to lose weight? Diet options ranged from A (Atkins) to Z (Zone) and private company programs from A (Awaken 180) to W (Weight Watchers). All claimed dramatic successes.

But all almost certainly fail over time. Research suggests that up to 97% of people regain their weight within about 3 years.[1] Here, for example, is UCLA researcher Traci Mann summarizing her own group's study:

> You can initially lose 5 to 10 percent of your weight on any number of diets, but then the weight comes back. We found that the majority of people regained all the weight, plus more.[2]

I didn't want to be one of the failures.

My doctor offered a nutritionist referral, which I postponed; I didn't like the odds, hate scheduling medical appointments and feared entering the modern diet culture even under the guise of organized medicine.

Instead, I decided to try on my own. I figured I could achieve at least the same dismal long- term weight loss result myself and possibly do

---

[1] The Weight of the Evidence, Harriet Brown, Slate, March 24, 2015
https://slate.com/technology/2015/03/diets-do-not-work-the-thin-evidence-that-losing-weight-makes-you-healthier.html.

[2] Dieting Does Not Work, Stuart Wolpert, UCLA Newsroom, April 3, 2007
https://newsroom.ucla.edu/releases/Dieting-Does-Not-Work-UCLA-Researchers-7832

even better.

This book describes how.

My program isn't a unique, novel or brilliant but it's straightforward, practical and honest. It may work for you.

Just follow the steps, modify it to your own needs and give yourself time.

Me fit-and-healthy pre-weight loss

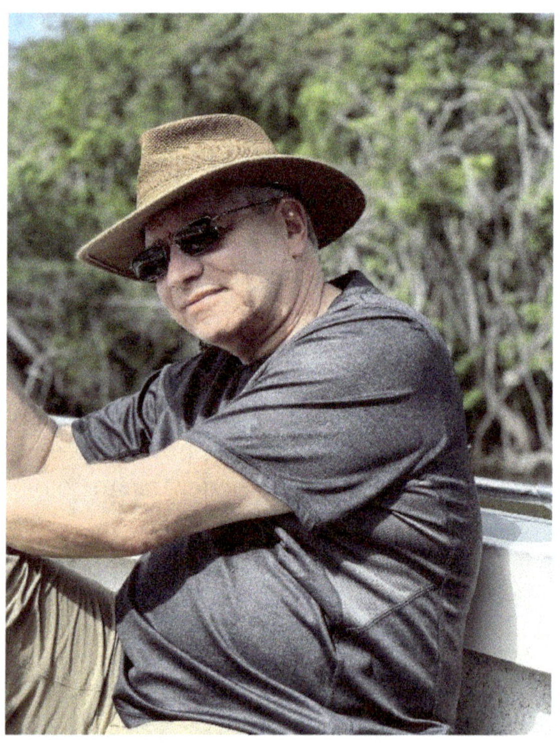

Introduction

I'm not a doctor, nutritionist, dietician or exercise physiologist. I have no medical training.

Instead, I'm an economist. I measure things. Weight loss strikes me as a measurement problem:

- If you eat more calories than you burn, you gain weight.
- If you eat fewer calories than you burn, you lose weight.
- As you eat less, your metabolism slows so you need to exercise more.

Sustained, long term weight loss also incorporates a fourth, behavioral consideration:

- Do this all slowly enough to develop new habits. That increases your chance of long-term success.

This program incorporates all those issues.

As background, I'm a 68-year-old, 73-inch-tall man. I weighed 225 pounds in my doctor's office on August 13, 2020.

I followed this program for 9 months and weighed 185 at my Sunday morning weigh-in April 4, 2021. I had lost 40 pounds over 36 weeks, about a pound per week on average.

It wasn't very difficult – more a task to accomplish than a mountain to climb - but I was hungry much of the time, especially at the beginning. That feeling dissipated as my new eating habits became ingrained and my body adjusted to its new setpoint.

I'm optimistic about long-term success, optimistic that my habits have changed enough to maintain my new weight for years to come. Cautiously optimistic that is, not blindly. We'll see. The future is a long time.

Gary Fradin

14

Step 1: Calculate your daily calorie needs.

There's a weight loss mantra 'eat 500 calories less each day and lose a pound a week'.

Maybe true – I don't know - but I needed a starting point. 500 calories less than what? No idea. I hadn't tracked my previous consumption.

I initially tried cutting cream from my morning coffee and dessert from lunch and dinner. But I didn't use the same amount of cream every day. Nor did I eat dessert every day but when I did, the type and size varied. Did that cut 500 calories? No idea.

I tried eating smaller portions. Small enough? Too small? Again, no idea. I only knew that I felt hungry. I worried that if I felt hungry without seeing results, I'd get frustrated and stop.

I needed a plan.

Instead of eating 500 calories less than some unknown number, I decided to calculate how many calories I *should* eat each day, a specific number, to lose a pound a week.

I googled 'calories per day to lose weight' and found lots of websites that base their estimates on age, height, weight, gender and daily activity level. Most suggested roughly the same amount – 2300 calories per day to lose a pound a week from that 225 pound starting point. (Your own amount will vary.)

The agreement among websites gave me a reasonable degree of confidence.

A sample calorie per day estimator
with my own data inserted [3]

| Age | 68 | ages 15 - 80 |

Gender ● male ○ female

| Height | 6 feet | 1 inches |

| Weight | 225 | pounds |

Activity Level

○ Basal Metabolic Rate (BMR)

○ Little or no exercise

○ Exercise 1-3 times/week

○ Exercise 4-5 times/week

● Daily exercise or intense exercise 3-4 times/week

○ Intense exercise 6-7 times/week

○ Very intense exercise daily, or physical job

I aimed for 2200 calories per day, slightly below the 2300 estimate to allow for measurement errors.

Interestingly, 2200 calories per day isn't a starvation diet. Far from it. In fact, the US Department of Agriculture estimates that the average

---

[3] This one comes from calculator.net with my data inserted.

American consumed 2234 calories per day in 1970.[4] My 2200 calorie target simply mimicked America's pre-obesity food consumption level.

Two thoughts on eating according to your daily calorie estimates and watching the impact on your weight:

- Set reasonable weight loss goals – neither too fast nor too much – to avoid frustration.
- Weigh yourself on the same scale, at the same time, every week. This generates the most consistent data, necessary to keep you on track. I choose Sunday mornings, first thing. Those are the weights I show in the **Results** section.

I started thinking 'if I can get down to 215, I'll be successful'. Then, upon reaching 215, I wondered about losing another 5 pounds. Then I aimed for 200, a nice round number. Then 195, a 30-pound loss and enough to write a book. Maybe others could benefit from this program?

But losing 40 pounds sounded better than 30, so I aimed for 185. That's where I ended, a weight that feels good, my doctor says is appropriate and is comfortably sustainable. I've held constant for 6 months and expect to for many more.

Remember that my initial goal wasn't 185. It was 215. Try to define success for yourself as a goal you can reasonably reach in a relatively short period, something that will make you feel proud. Then let the future take care of itself as you gain confidence through success.

---

[4] Wells and Buzby, US Food Consumption Up 16% Since 1970, Economic Research Service US Department of Agriculture, November 1, 2005
https://www.ers.usda.gov/amber-waves/2005/november/us-food-consumption-up-16-percent-since-1970/

Gary Fradin

Step 2: Divide your daily calorie target into 3 meals and a snack.

I used this rule-of-thumb for my initial 2200 calorie per day program.

- Breakfast - 400 calories (approx. 18% of total daily calories)
- Lunch - 600 calories (27%)
- Dinner - 800 calories (36%)
- Snacks or dessert - 400 calories. You can add these to your breakfast, lunch or dinner.

Your own calorie target and meal amounts will differ based on your own age, height, weight, gender, physical activity level and desired weight loss speed.

You'll find calorie estimates for specific foods on packages or online. Simply google 'calories in a medium potato' or 'calories in a cup of blueberries' or whatever. It's easy and close enough for our purposes.

Meal timing: I ate according to the clock throughout this program and expect to in the future:

Breakfast time

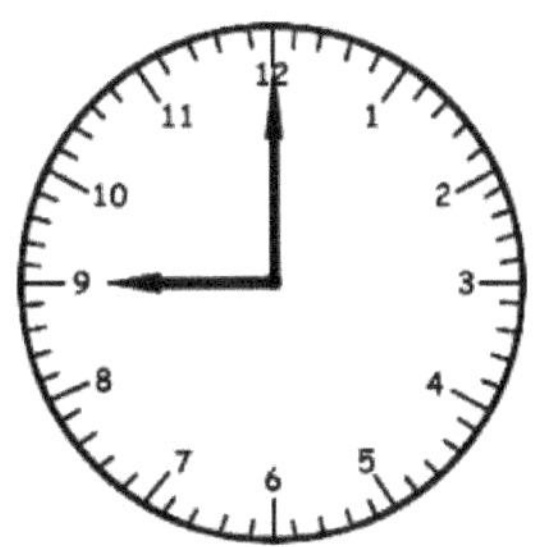

Lunch time

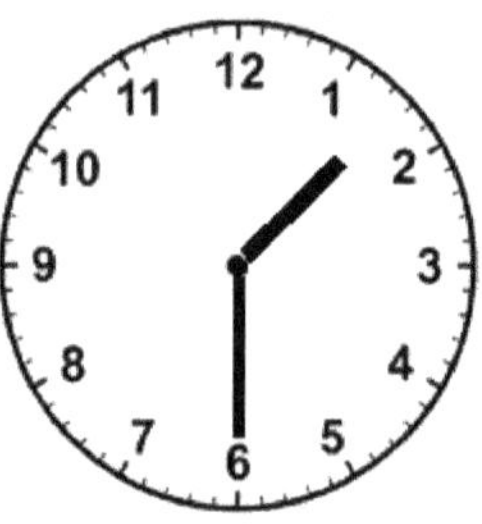

Dinner time

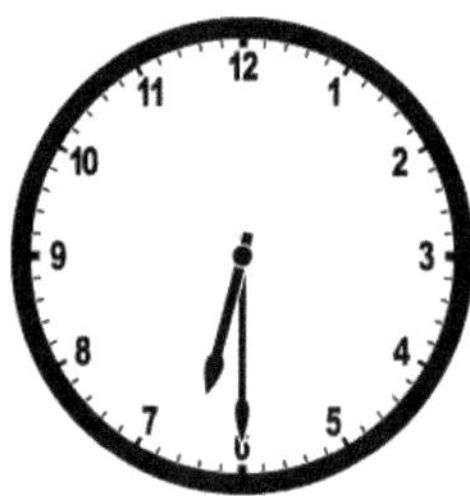

Try not to eat whenever you feel hungry because those feelings come and go. Stick to the clock. It's honest, reliable and will keep you on track.

Aim to develop **habits** like mealtimes and food combinations.

The more routine and predictable you make this program, the more likely you are to stay on it and succeed.

Food choices: I learned several things through trial and error about my own reaction to food groups. You probably will too.

First, I feel full after eating fruits and vegetables probably because of their high fiber and water contents. I eat lots of both these days.

Second, I feel full *longer* after eating fat and protein like nuts. My go-to snack these days is almond, peanut or cashew butter spread on a sliced apple or banana. All natural, no additives. Very filling.

Third, I prefer healthy food tastes. I look forward to my English muffin, peanut butter and banana breakfast today as enthusiastically as I had previously anticipated pancakes with syrup or eggs with bacon, sausage and toast.

In fact, I no longer want those overly-sweet, overly-salty, overly-filling, low-fiber meals, not only because they're so high in in calories but because they make me feel lousy afterward. They sit like a rock in my stomach and leave me stuffed and thirsty, then surprisingly hungry relatively quickly.

My breakfast taste evolution
Too sweet

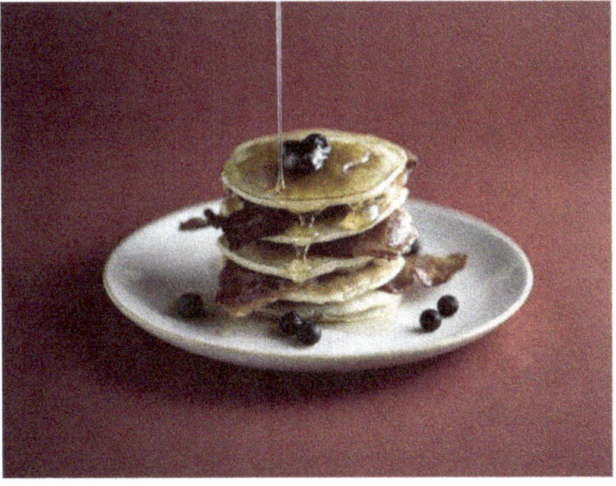

Pancake stack with bacon & syrup = about 700 calories

Too salty

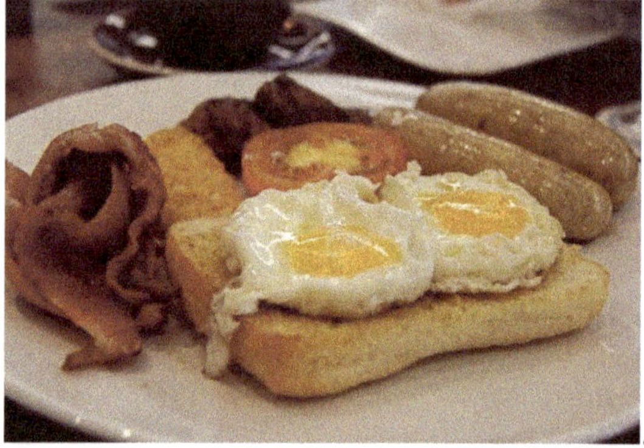

2 eggs, bacon, sausages, toast & tomato = about 600 calories

Just right

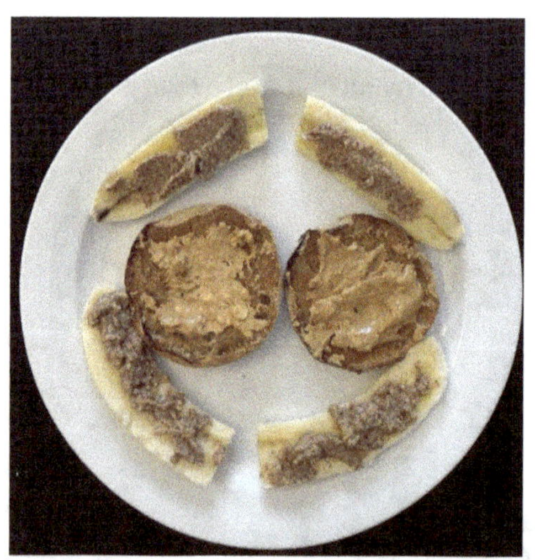

Peanut butter on a toasted English muffin
with almond butter on a banana = about 400 calories.

Fourth, I don't miss calorie-rich tastes, things like cream in my
morning coffee, cheese and crackers between meals or chocolate cake
after dinner. I now prefer blueberries, raspberries or strawberries for

dessert, sometimes with a drop of honey on top. Berries are sweet and delicious, and I feel good after eating them.

Plus I don't get that sugary thirst like after eating cookies or cake.

My experiences mirror recommendations from 2 thoughtful sources. Michael Pollan, New York Times contributor, best-selling author, and Berkeley professor famously advises people to "Eat food. Not too much. Mostly plants." Consider each phrase.

> **"Eat food"** means real, identifiable farm products like fruits, vegetables, whole grains, meat and fish. Avoid ingredients you can't pronounce and foods your grandmother wouldn't recognize.

> **"Not too much"** means stick to your daily calorie limit.

> **"Mostly plants"** means lots of fruit and vegetables.

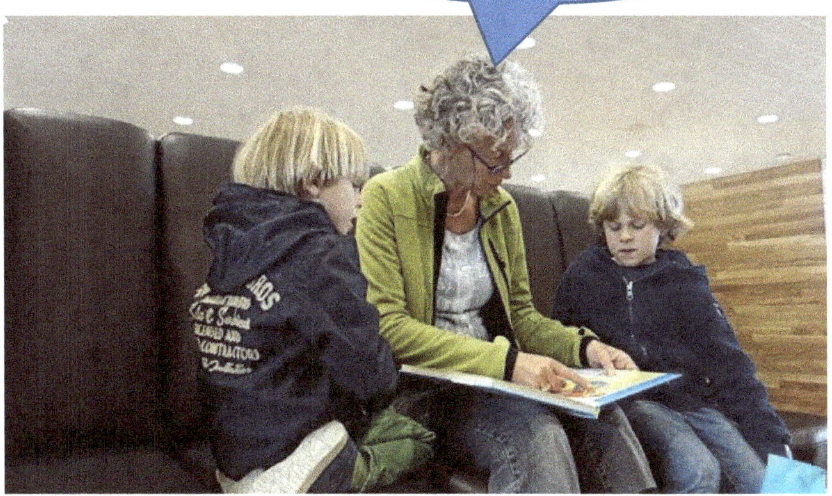

Grandmother giving time honored advice.

Next, the Canadian Food Plate, photo below, suggests the proportion of each food group – plants, grains and proteins – to eat daily. Remember that nuts, beans and legumes count as proteins.

About half your plate should be fruits and veggies, a quarter protein both animal and vegetable, and another quarter whole grains.

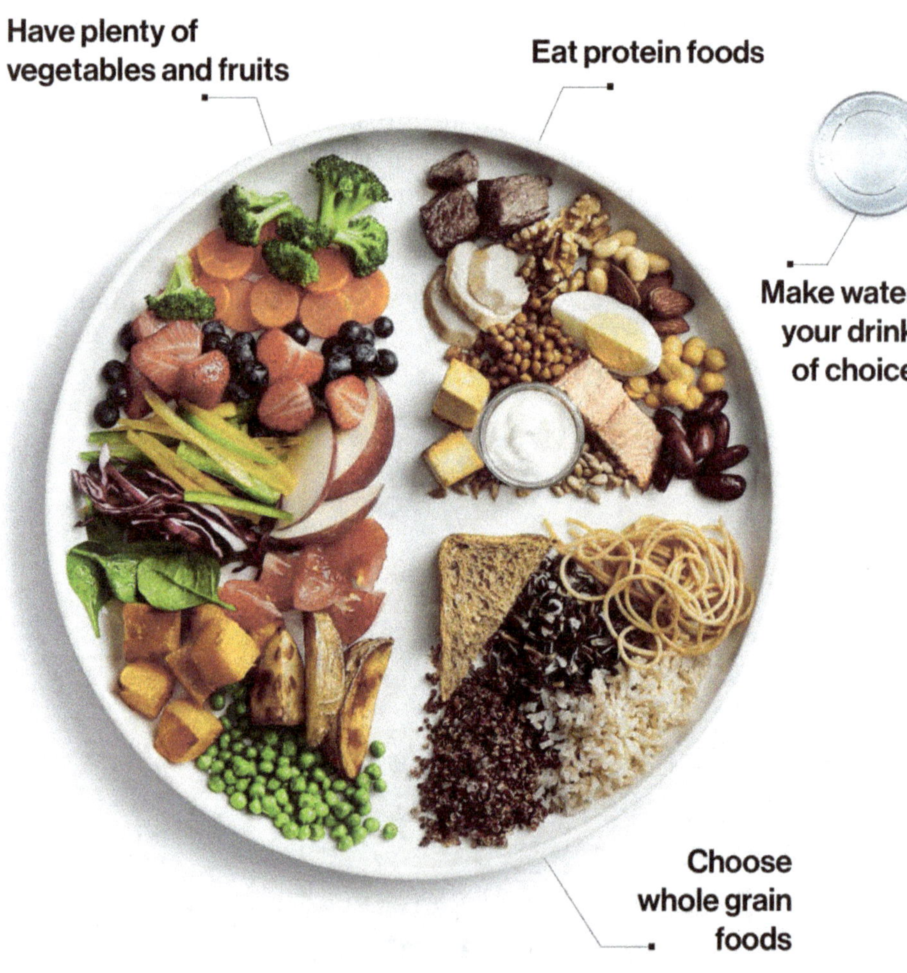

Eat food. Not too much. Mostly plants.

Tastes and habits: When people say, 'I can't drink coffee without milk and sugar' or 'I can't eat a sandwich without potato chips', I wonder if they remember what got them into their overweight situation in the first place.

Changing eating habits is a process, both challenging and rewarding. The good news is that you really can change.

The bad news is it takes time. Most people require at least 2 months for a new taste preference to become fully automatic though some people take up to 8 months according to research.[5]

I needed the full 8 months. And then some.

Understand and accept this. Give yourself time to change your habits and develop new eating routines.

This relatively lengthy process may suggest why our modern diet industry so often fails people. It operates within two mutually exclusive constraints.

- First, it has to deliver weight loss results quickly enough that people don't drop out and post negative reviews online.

- But second, long term sustained weight loss and new habit creation takes a long time.

You can't generate fast results slowly! That's why I didn't want to get involved with it. I wanted a program without commercial or time pressure.

---

[5] Grohol, Need to Form a New Habit? Give Yourself At Least 66 Days, PsychCentral, October 7, 2018 https://psychcentral.com/blog/need-to-form-a-new-habit-66-days ; UCL News August 9, 2009 Interview with Phillippa Lally https://www.ucl.ac.uk/news/2009/aug/how-long-does-it-take-form-habit

A practical suggestion to help you change your eating habits.

Write down your calorie consumption after **everything** you eat. This includes the half cookie in the afternoon, the glass of wine before dinner and 'just a tase' of your favorite dessert in the evening.

You'll see examples in the **Write Everything Down** section.

My meals and snacks don't feel finished these days until I complete this form. I expect this habit to continue for life because it works.

Hunger. Eating fewer calories per day makes you hungry. That's simply reality. I learned to differentiate three types of hunger.

Hunger as not feeling completely full. I had previously enjoyed eating until I was 'pleasantly satisfied'. I don't get that feeling anymore.

Instead, I feel 'full enough' these days, not exactly hungry but not completely full either. I could happily eat an additional muffin at breakfast, a bigger sandwich at lunch or an extra helping at dinner. But I don't.

I've learned to embrace feeling 'full enough' when I reach my calorie limit per meal. It's my new normal, my new habit. Today it feels right.

You can adapt to this new feeling too. Just give yourself time. And remember your goal.

Hunger as deprivation, actual physical need, sometimes called 'belly hunger' as opposed to 'head hunger', below.

I wasn't worried about physical deprivation as long as I ate every 4 – 5 hours. I knew that my 2200 calorie per day program was sufficient for good health - the 1970 era US food experience proved that. Two hundred million Americans ate that way every day. End of story as far as I was concerned.

Some people, of course, might have special nutrition or health issues. I can't speak to those. Still not a doctor.

Belly hunger differs from head hunger. Head hunger goes away when you think about something else. Belly hunger does not.

Try this thought experiment to understand the difference: visualize a delicious burger or juicy steak or moist chocolate cake or juicy mango. Imagine the taste. Picture it. Anticipate the sensation as you bite in.

Hold that thought. Feel hungry? It's head hunger.

Now think of an IRS audit or root canal surgery. Visualize it. Hold onto it. Lose the hungry feeling?

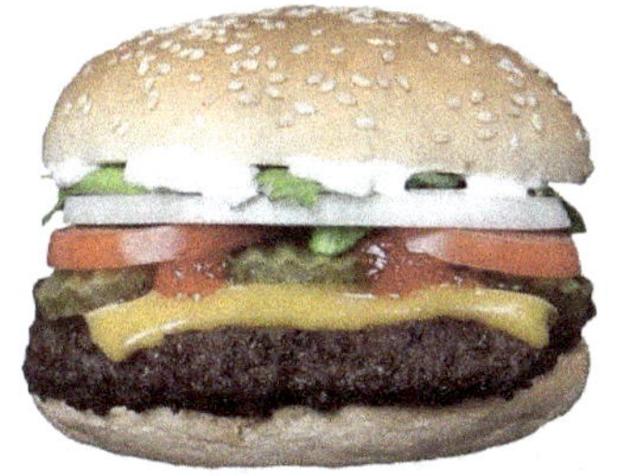

Causes head hunger

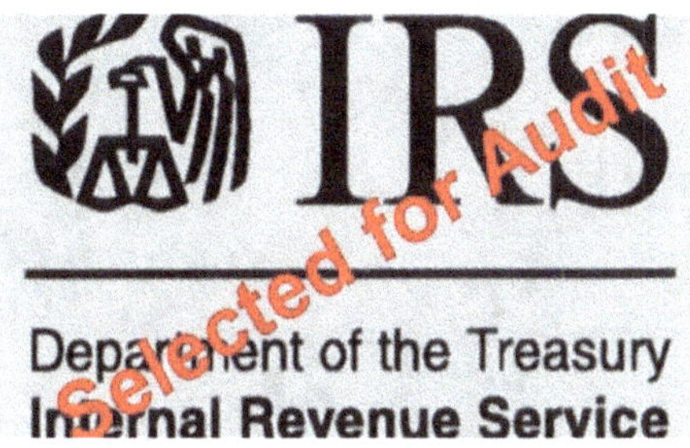

Removes head hunger

Head hunger is a mental state. You can feel it equally few hours after either a big or small meal. When you feel it, think about something else. Easier said than done of course.

Three tricks help me:

- I threw out all junk food from our house. Too tempting. Out-of-sight, out-of-mind.

- When I feel hungry between meals, I force myself to _do_ something: take a walk, call a friend, work on my computer, prepare for a business meeting, take a drive… something that actively engages my mind. I find that passively watching TV or reading a book doesn't work, but that's just me. You might have a different experience. Experiment!

- When I watch TV in the evening – after dinner and dessert – I try to do something with my hands like hold my cell phone and read news updates. Some people knit or draw. This additional activity keeps your focus away from bodily sensations like hunger. Maybe that trick will work for you too.

I also drink lots of water.

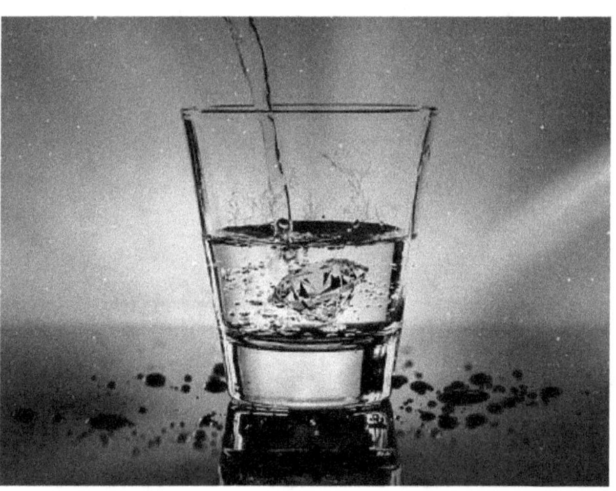

Quick rule-of-thumb about water. Divide your weight in pounds by 2. That's how many ounces of water to drink each day.

In my case, 185 pounds / 2 = 92 ounces of water. Close enough for government work. Check with your doc to be sure.

It's a Goldilocks principle: not too little, not too much, just right.

A Real Life Head Hunger Experience

I returned from a walk one day around 1:15, tired and hungry.

As I began to prepare lunch, my oldest son called. He had just finished a job interview and wanted to describe it. Fine, I listened – that's what fathers do. My lunch could wait a few minutes.

Then, as I opened a bag of vegetables, a client called wanting to prepay for an upcoming program. Ok, first rule of thumb for self-employed businesspeople like me: when someone offers to pay, say yes. Lunch could wait a few more minutes.

While processing his payment, my computer beeped. A different client emailed to propose a new, potentially lucrative program. Could we speak about it in a day or two?

My mind raced with preparation issues. Second rule of thumb for small business owners: when you think of something, write it down. I jotted down notes, reviewed some old files and began to think through our upcoming phone conversation.

Suddenly it was 3:15. Two hours had passed since I got home feeling hungry. Somehow I had forgotten to eat.

It was head hunger after all. No big deal.

Food costs. Vegetables, per calorie, cost more than most other food groups due to various food subsidy and tax programs. Here are some retail examples per 100 calories:[6]

---

[6] I googled most of these on March 15, 2021 and looked in our refrigerator for others. I simply divided the cost per unit – pound or bag – by the total number of calories contained.

Food	Cost / unit	Cost/100 calories [7]
93% Lean Ground Beef	$9.19 per pound	$1.33
Purdue Boneless Chicken Breast	$10.39 per 1.5 lb package	$1.38
Signature Farms Broccoli and Cauliflower	$5.99 per 28 ounce bag	$2.66
Fresh Express Veggie Lovers Salad	$2.99 per bag	$5.75
Red On-the-Vine Tomatoes	$3.49 per pound	$4.26

Healthy food costs more! Be prepared for a food budget increase.

Restaurants pose a problem for calorie restricted diets. Here are four suggestions that might help:

- Split a main course with someone and complement each portion with a side salad.

- Stick with salads and protein toppings. Careful with the dressing. This option might make the restaurant experience less special, but it will make your calorie intake more predictable and manageable.

- Ask the restaurant to bring a doggie-bag containing half of your meal **when they serve it**. I find this works better than attempting to estimate and eat half first, then asking for a doggie bag later.

---

[7] I used 100 calories rather than per calorie because the individual calorie costs involve portions of a penny. Too confusing.

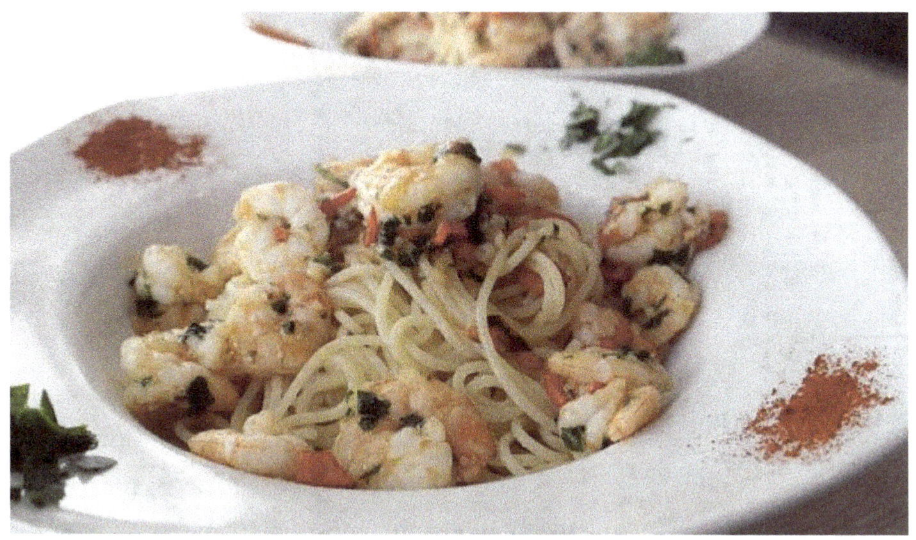

Ask for half in a doggie-bag *when you order*.

- Pay attention to drinks, both alcoholic and non. Wine has about 120 calories per glass, beer 150, gin and tonic 170, Long Island iced tea 280 and Margaritas up to 450.[8] Coca-Cola classic has 140 calories per 12 ounces, orange juice about 110 per cup and chocolate milk about 200. Those all count toward your daily total.

---

[8] Best and Worst Booze While Dieting, Carolyn Williams on cookinglight.com
https://www.cookinglight.com/healthy-living/weight-loss/best-alcohol-drink-on-diet

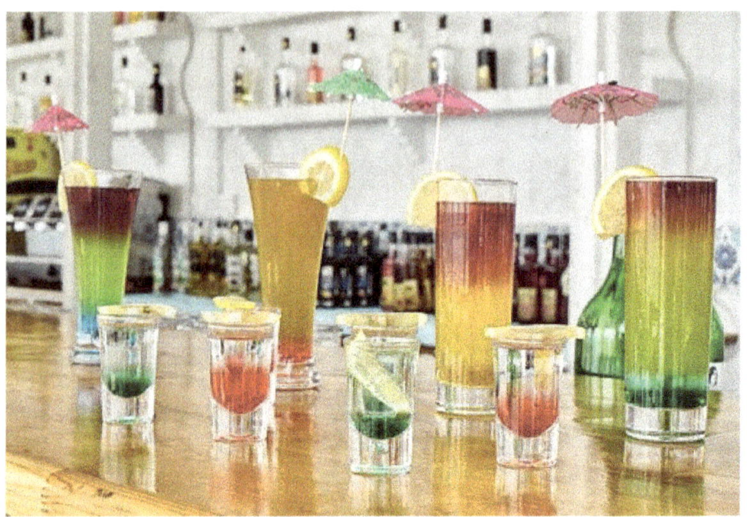

These calories all count

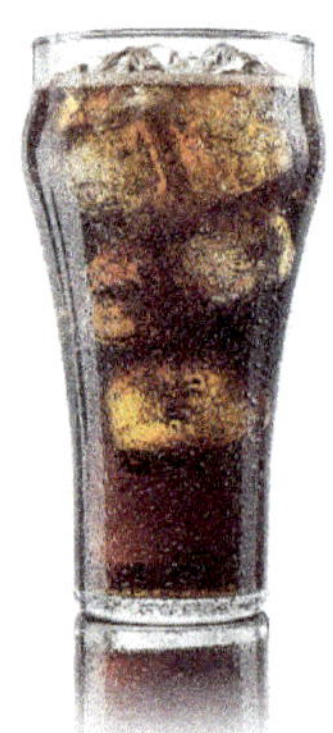

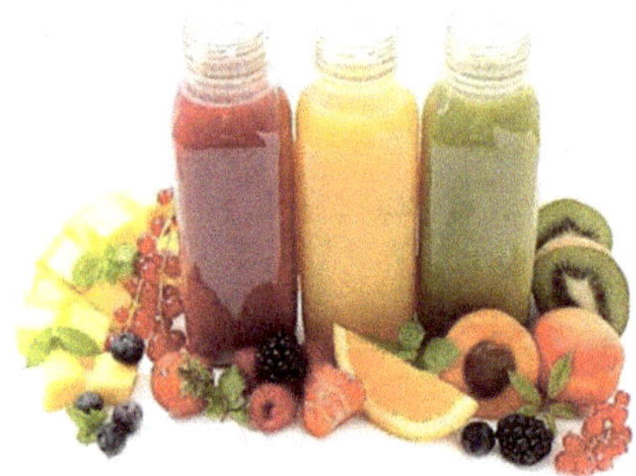

These too

See which of these restaurant suggestions works best for you. Maybe you can discover another.

Cheating: Try not to. You'll only sabotage your progress and depress yourself at your next weekly weigh in. Be honest with your measurements and anticipate that you'll be on this program for several months at least, maybe for life (maintenance period).

Using food as a reward: Try to change your thinking from 'I did a good job (at something), so I'll reward myself with ice cream' or chocolate cake or nachos and beer or some other tasty treat.

Try to think of 'doing a good job' and 'eating' as unrelated activities.

- 'Do a good job' because it's the right thing to do and makes you feel good.

- 'Eating wisely' is also the right thing to do and makes you feel good.

- But 'eating unwisely' *isn't* the right thing to do because it generally makes you feel badly, either physically, emotionally, or intellectually ('why did I just eat that?').

Doing the wrong thing to reward yourself after doing the right thing doesn't work. I know from experience.

****

I invented some recipes, unexpected food combinations that satisfied me. Several became my new habits. If you like any, use them. Feel free to invent your own!

Breakfast

Toasted English muffin with peanut butter plus a banana with almond butter. I eat this most frequently, perhaps 5 times per week. Cut a whole wheat English muffin (100 calories) in half and toast both halves. Then spread one tablespoon of salt-free peanut butter – about 100 calories – onto the 2 halves, about half a tablespoon per half. I don't add jam because I don't like sweet tastes for breakfast, but that's just me.

Then cut a ripe banana, about 100 calories, in half and spread one tablespoon of almond butter – about 100 calories - onto it, again half a tablespoon per half. I prefer almond butter to peanut butter with bananas but again, my own preference.

Poached eggs on oatmeal. Instead of 2 scrambled eggs and 2 pieces of toast for breakfast, I sometimes substitute 2 poached eggs over oatmeal with a splash of ketchup, again my own taste preference. Oatmeal instead of wheat, one grain for another. Make it thick. One-third cup of steel oats is 170 calories, two jumbo eggs total 180.

Sometimes I add tomato slices or steamed broccoli. Tasty. Other times I melt Swiss cheese into the oatmeal, then put one egg on top. Delicious!

Plenty of other breakfast options exist within that original 400 calorie constraint. You're only limited by your imagination.

Lunch

I often eat leftovers for lunch, generally vegetables with some protein and fruit for dessert. Sometimes I add peanuts, cashews or butter beans - I really like butter beans - depending on our refrigerator's contents. Remember to estimate your calories honestly when you do this.

Here are some creative combinations that I enjoyed.

Tuna fish sandwich with pickles and a chocolate banana smoothie. I use chunk light tuna, only 90 calories per can, oilier than solid white so requiring less mayonnaise; add about ½ tablespoon, 50 calories. Then 2 slices of bread @ 100 calories each, a tomato slice and lettuce with a side of pickles for a 360 calorie, filling sandwich. Maybe add a splash of mustard (!) for flavor.

Then, assuming your taste buds require (mine generally do), make a frozen banana smoothie. One cup of skim milk (100 calories), a banana (another 100) and 2 tablespoons of Ovaltine (40 calories). I prefer Ovaltine to other chocolate syrups, but again, that's just me. Total about 240 calories, making your tuna sandwich plus smoothie a tasty 600 calorie lunch.

Beans or mussels in tomato sauce over steamed vegetables. One 8-ounce packet of frozen mussels (I use PanaPesca) contains 175 calories; 3 cups of broad beans about 150 calories. One cup of tomato or marinara sauce has about 120 calories depending on the brand. Put this modified bolognaise sauce over steamed zucchini, broccoli or cauliflower and sprinkle with parmesan cheese for a delicious and filling 300 calorie lunch. Enjoy a couple pieces of fruit for dessert.

I sometimes substitute chicken, garbanzo beans or left-over steak.

And I sometimes, though rarely, put this over a cup of pasta, about 200 calories.

Plenty of options to try.

A word about vegetables and salad. Per volume, vegetables contain fewer calories than most other foods. It's hard to overeat spinach or broccoli!

Try mixing three cups of raw spinach (25 calories) with a cup of raw beets (45 calories), a large tomato (25 calories), left over veggies from your refrigerator and any other vegetables you have on-hand. Then top with your favorite cheese, nuts or protein.

Careful with the dressing though. I limit myself to 1 tablespoon, generally of Italian or Greek dressing, about 75 calories depending on the brand. Sometimes I make my own, mixing olive oil, vinegar and mustard or horseradish. Sometimes I just splash red wine vinegar over my salad. It's a taste I've come to enjoy.

I eat salads regularly but not daily because I prefer grilled vegetables to raw. Personal preference again.

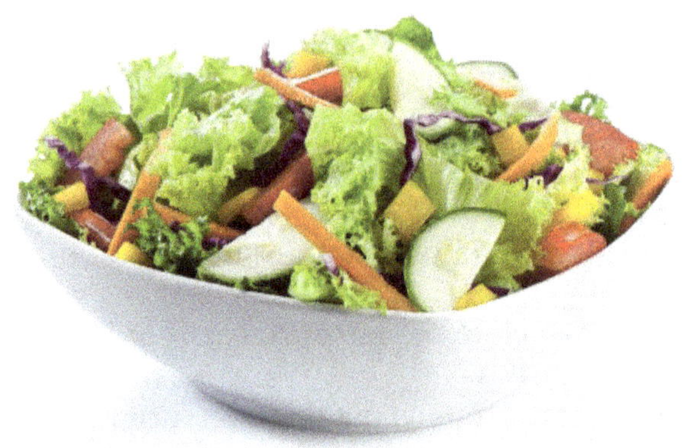

Many days

A word about fruit. I normally eat at least 3 pieces of fruit every day in addition to my frequent morning banana. I'm partial to apples, oranges, strawberries, raspberries and blueberries. We're not, in my family, big melon, pineapple or mango people but if we were, I'd include those too. It's a matter of taste again.

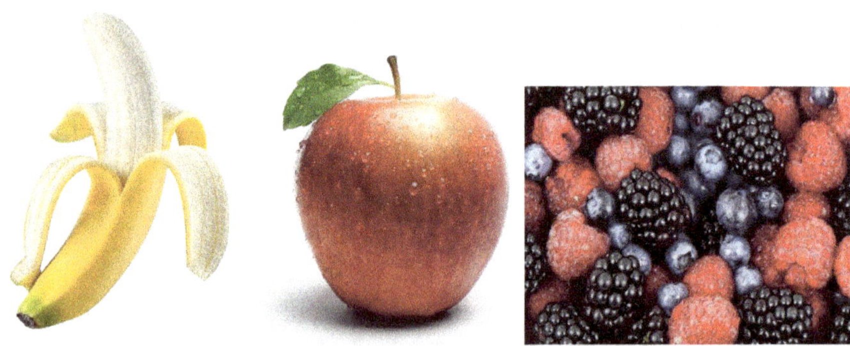

Everyday

Dinner

We enjoy broiled vegetables frequently during the winter and grilled veg in the summer, generally broccoli, cauliflower, green beans, asparagus, or eggplant. I char them slightly and sometimes sprinkle lightly with salad dressing. ('Lightly' means about a tablespoon per pound of veg.)

We typically eat this as a side dish with grilled meat, chicken or fish, most often fish. Sometimes my wife and I split a sweet potato too, about 80 calories per half. That adds natural sweetness to the meal.

Remember to control your portions! Steak has more calories per pound than chicken; salmon more than white fish.

Tomato sauce with turkey or beans and vegetables. This becomes a stand-alone bolognaise type stew; no pasta required. We use low fat ground turkey, a low calorie / low salt pasta sauce (read the labels) and add broccoli, cauliflower, peas, onions, mushrooms, peppers or fresh tomatoes. Then flavor with red wine.

We sometimes substitute butter beans for the turkey.

One issue with this meal: estimating calories accurately, especially leftovers. I generally add up all the calories in the entire batch, then estimate portion size – a quarter, a third, etc. Close enough for our purposes. Overestimating your portion today leads to underestimating it tomorrow or vice versa.

I then label the leftover calories in the fridge because I forget otherwise.

Baked feta and vegetables. Cut a block of feta cheese into 300 calorie chunks then bake or broil with red onions and cherry tomatoes. Sprinkle lightly with Greek salad dressing. Add a glass of chilled white wine, about 100 calories.

We sometimes substitute tofu for feta. Same idea, different flavor.

Homemade oatmeal muesli, a sweet, Swiss-themed change from veggies and protein. Mix 1/2 cup of steel cut oatmeal (255 calories), ½ cup of unsalted cashews or peanuts (320 cal.) or almonds (414 cal), a cup of blueberries (85 cal.), a cup of strawberries (50 cal.) and a banana (100 cal.). Total about 800 calories depending on your specific ingredients. Top with yogurt or honey, another 70 calories or sprinkled coconut. Eat hot or cold.

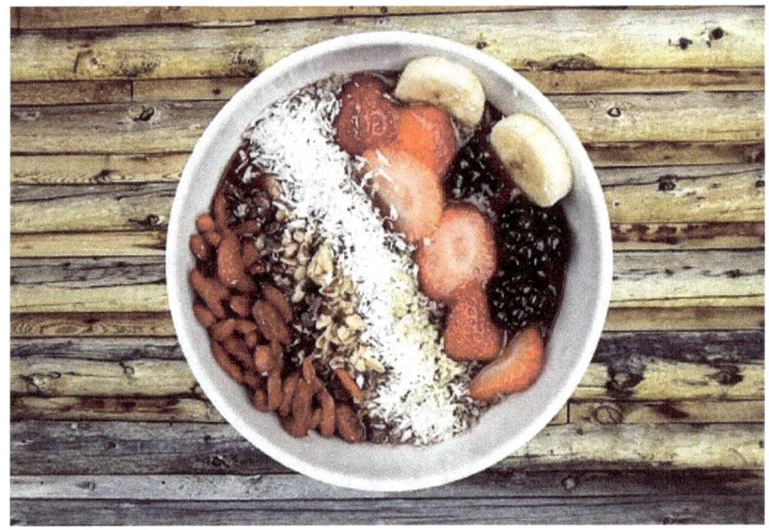

A delicious muesli dinner

Snacks and Deserts

Some of my favorite quick-and-easy snacks include:

- Baked sliced apples with cinnamon. About 100 cal. per apple.

- Blueberries or raspberries. 85 cal. per cup each + 1 tablespoon honey, 70 cal. equals 155 calories total.

- Yogurt with Ovaltine. ½ cup fat free, sugar free yogurt, 60 cal. + 2 tablespoons of Ovaltine, 40 cal. = 100 calorie version of chocolate mousse. OK, not exactly mousse but it's pretty good. I sometimes double this if I'm ahead on my daily calories. I eat this pretty frequently because I'm a bona-fide chocaholic.

- Sliced apple (100 cal.) with almond butter or cashew butter (90 cal. per tablespoon), 190 calorie total. As satisfying as a heavily sugared peanut butter cookie and you feel much better afterwards. This has become my go-to snack.

- Nut and dried fruit trail mix. Combine chopped dried dates, figs, apricots and raisins with crushed almonds, cashews and peanuts, then flavor with Frangelico, Drambuie, Grand Marnier or your own preferred liquor. Divide into 150 or 200 calorie portions and store in individual plastic bags. Modify per your own taste. This is a particularly good snack for road trips and airplane rides.

You'll invent your own recipes. Write everything down so you remember which worked best for you.

40

Step 3: Go for a daily brisk walk.
or get some other form of daily exercise

Our metabolisms slow down as we eat fewer calories. To counter this, exercise every day.

I normally enjoy a brisk daily walk, equal emphasis on **brisk** and **daily**. 'Brisk' means you can just barely keep a conversation going. Walk with a friend to find your own speed using this metric. (Check with your doctor to make sure you're healthy enough first.)

**Our frighteningly unfashionable hero in his
winter walking outfit, 2021**

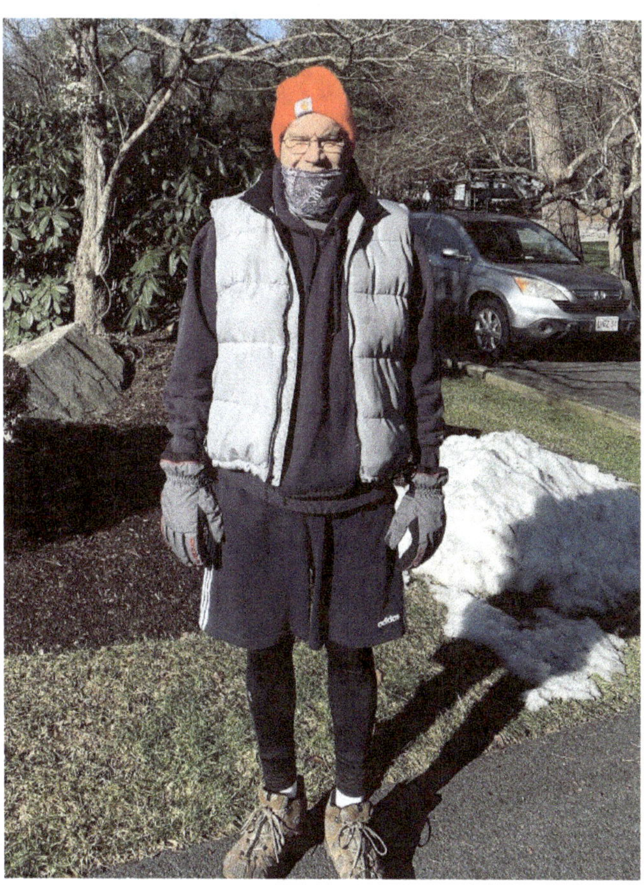

I average about 420 minutes – 7 hours – of brisk walking per week. I measure minutes of exercise per day instead of steps or total walking distance to allow for swimming, bike riding, exercise classes, weightlifting, skating, cross country skiing or other exercise forms.

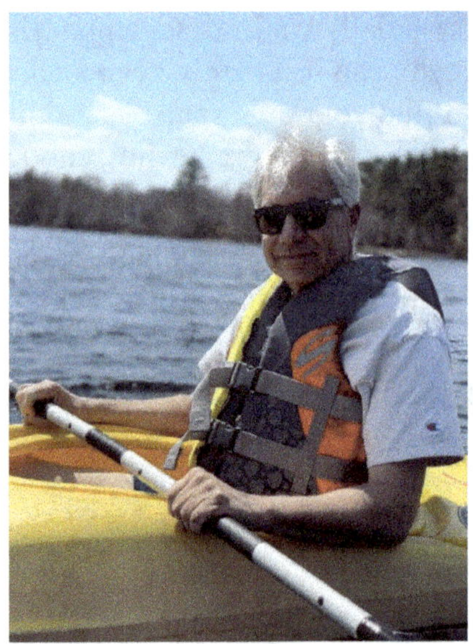

Kayaking counts too

Interestingly, both the US Centers for Disease Control and British National Health Service recommend <u>at least</u> 150 minutes per week of brisk exercise for everyone. More is better. Those 420 minutes of weekly exercise helped keep my metabolism from slowing down as I ate fewer calories.

Daily exercise – generally walking in my case - like everything else in this book becomes a habit. You miss it on days you don't go. Allow yourself time for this habit to develop and for exercise to become your daily routine.

I like to measure both my daily exercise time and walking distance. The goal is to maintain at least, and hopefully increase, both. Various smart phone apps can help.

One day, early in this program, I walked 4 miles in 70 minutes, about 17.5 minutes per mile, finishing tired and certain I couldn't go farther or faster. Six months later, on a mid-February walk, I averaged 15:30 per mile for 5 miles, equally certain that I couldn't go faster … but pretty sure, this time, that I could go farther. (I actually went 7 miles a week later though at a slower 16:30 pace.)

One trick that keeps me motivated, even enthusiastic about walking every day: I listen to novels, generally long ones that keep me engaged. I prefer historical fiction and mysteries but again, personal preference.

I've walked with Winston Churchill during the Blitz of London, young Nigerian intellectuals as they navigate life, Sherlock Holmes, seafaring merchants, unscrupulous criminals, clever detectives and many others. I look forward each day to reconnecting with my audio friends and often – oddly – feel sad when each book ends. Listening while walking has become another habit, one that I increasingly enjoy.

Confessionary addendum: I know that I should add strength training to my exercise regime. I keep meaning to start but, truth be told, I never enjoyed lifting weights or doing sit-ups. Maybe I'll start tomorrow.

Doubtful.

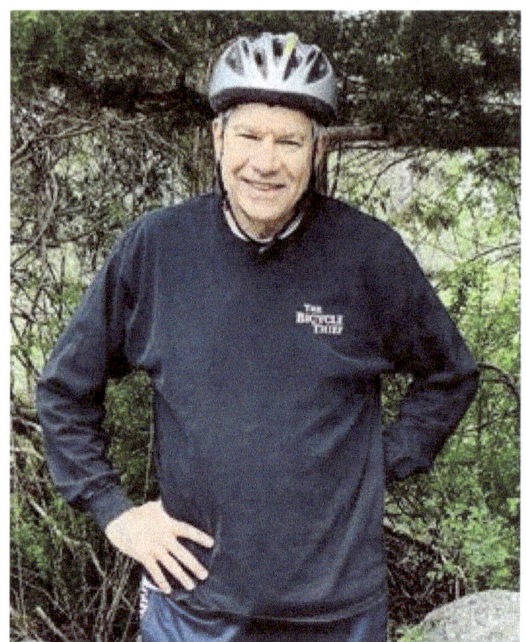

**Bike riding also counts
but don't listen to novels while you ride!**

Step 4: Write *everything* down.

Write down your food consumption after every meal and snack, and your exercise time (or whichever exercise metric you choose) every day. That keeps you on track to achieve your goals.

While apps exist for this, I prefer the forms below. Personal choice again. Completing them becomes another habit. It takes a minute or so. I expect to continue this for years since I plan to stay in the 180 pound weight range for a long time.

Remember to write down the little taste of dessert, small glass of wine and nibble in the afternoon. They all count. So does the ketchup on your burger.

As you write things down, you'll notice patterns and adjust. Absent this written log, you'll have more trouble noticing trends and identifying causes.

Weigh-ins: I weigh myself first thing every Sunday morning. That's my 'official' weight though I confess to checking more frequently. I worry, slightly, that daily weigh-ins will drive me crazy, or, more likely, my wife. I'm already obsessive enough!

Beware of salt and water retention at your weigh-ins. Eating a salty evening meal – feta cheese or pasta sauce for example – can increase my weight by 2 to 3 pounds the next morning. Factor this into your calculations and, perhaps more importantly, watch your daily salt consumption. Harder to do than say unfortunately.

Track your daily calories: Use the attached simple form. You'll see patterns emerge pretty quickly. Plus this will keep you from overeating in response to head-hunger.

I've inserted a week of meals simply as an example using my original 2200 calorie per day target. You can set up these forms in Excel very easily and design your own meals.

Day	Breakfast	Lunch	Dinner	Snack(s)	Total/Day
Sun	Eng Muffin (100) Pnut butter (100) Banana (100) Almond butter (100) Total 400	Salad bag (50) Tomato (30) Chicken left overs (300) Italian dressing (75) Apple (100) Total 555	Turkey stew (ground turkey, pasta sauce and veg) (750) Salad and dressing (100) Pineapple (120) Total 970	3 Clementine (105) Yogurt & Ovaltine (100) Blueberries & honey (150) Total 355	2280
Mon	Oatmeal (170) 2 jumbo eggs (180) Ketchup (20) Total 370	Cauliflower left overs (75) Butter beans (150) Dressing (75) Chicken (150) Apple & cashew butr (190) Total 640	Salmon (300) Broccoli (100) Salad (50) & Dressing (75) Wine (100) 3 clementine (105) Total 730	Banana & almond buttr (100) Blueberries & honey (150) Yogurt & ovaltine (200) Total 450	2190
Tues	Eng Muffin (100) Pnut butter (100) Banana (100) Almond butter (100) Total 400	Broad beans (200) Steamed veg (150) Dressing (75) 2 sm oranges(180) Total 605	Cod & panko (450) Salad & beans (200) Dressing (75) 1 slice bread (100) Total 825	Blueberries & Activia (220) Orange (100) Apple (100) Total 420	2250
Wed	Eng Muffin (100) Pnut butter (100) Banana (100) Almond butter (100) Total 400	Impossible burger (270) 2 x Bread (200) L & T, mustard, pickle (30) Apple (100) Total 600	Oatmeal (170) Cashews (320) 2 cups frozen fruit (140) Honey (70) Total 700	Baked apple & cinn (200) Yogurt & Ovaltine (200) Total 400	2100
Thurs	Eng Muffin	Tuna (90),	Swordfish	Apple (100)	

	(100) Pnut butter (100) Banana (100) Almond butter (100) Total 400	mayo (50) 2 x Bread (200) Pickles, L & T (40) Skim milk & banana (200) Ovaltine (40) Total 640	(400) Broccoli (200) Green beans (100) Dressing (75) Blueberries (85) Total 860	Orange (100) 2 x Clem (70) Total 270	2170
Fri	Oatmeal (170) 2 jumbo eggs (180) Ketchup (20) Tomato (30) Total 400	Broccoli (100) Green means (50) Swordfish (200) Dressing (50) Pear & orange (200) Total 600	Baked feta (300) Tomatoes, onions (50) Broccoli (100) Potato (200) Wine (100) Total 750	Blueberries & honey (180) Yogurt & Oval (200) Clem (100) Total 480	2230
Sat	Oatmeal (170) Swiss cheese (100) 1 egg (90) Ketchup (20) Total 380	Tuna (90), mayo (50) Eng muffin (100) Pickles, L & T (40) Skim milk & banana (200) Ovaltine (40), Apple (100) Total 580	Beans (200) Rice (200) 1/3 cup cashews (250) Salad and dressing (150) Blueberries (100) Total 900	Baked apple & cinn (200) Yogurt & Oval (100) Orange (100) Total 400	2260

Exercise Use this form to track your daily exercise, total mileage or steps. If you track exercise minutes, focus on brisk walking minutes, the time your heart beats more quickly than normal, when you can just barely keep a conversation going.

You can modify this to track your daily walking steps, mileage or any other metric you choose. Just remember to exercise daily and write everything down.

Exercise minutes per day

	Sun	Mon	Tues	Wed	Thurs	Fri	Sat	Total
date								
date								
date								

Results

This program worked for me. It may also work for you.

If you decide to try, give it an honest effort. Stick with it for at least 6 months, long enough to develop new food habits.

Below, a sample of my own experience from October to December 2020, enough to make the point.

Weekly Food Consumption, Exercise and Weight Change

Week Ending Date	Average Calories Consumed per Day	Total Exercise Walking Minutes per Week	Sunday Morning Weight	Weight change, pounds, rounded
Oct 4	2120	465	207	
Oct 11	2020	535	206	-1
Oct 18	2230	465	204	-2
Oct 25	2110	550	203	-1
Nov 1	2300	360	202	-1
Nov 8	2019	475	201	-1
Nov 15	2087	455	200	-1
Nov 22	2657 (Thanksgiving)	580	198	-2
Nov 29	2069	540	199	+1
Dec 6	2157	320	196	-3
Dec 13	2452	485	195	-1

Dec 20	1999	340	197	+2
Dec 27	2400	410	196	-1
Jan 3, 2021	2332	600	195	-1
Averages over 14 weeks	2210	470		**-.9 lb. per week**

I hope you see how developing good habits can sustain your weight loss and subsequent weight maintenance.

My new habits – eating at set times, allocating half my plate to fruits and vegetables, portion control, and daily exercise – took months to develop but are now ingrained into my daily life. They've become my new normal.

I'm optimistic that they will continue for years into the future.

Before, 225 pounds

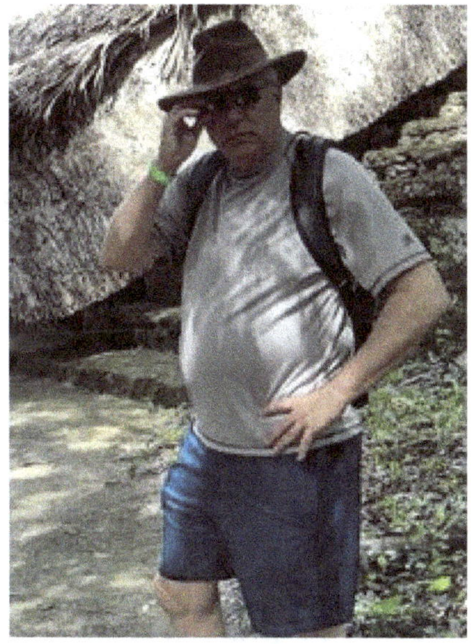

After, 185 pounds

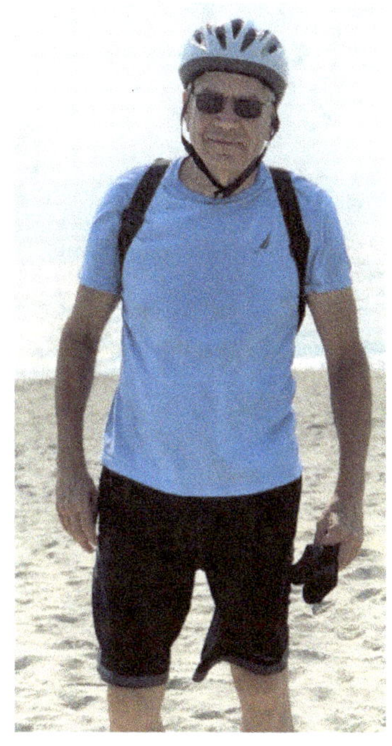

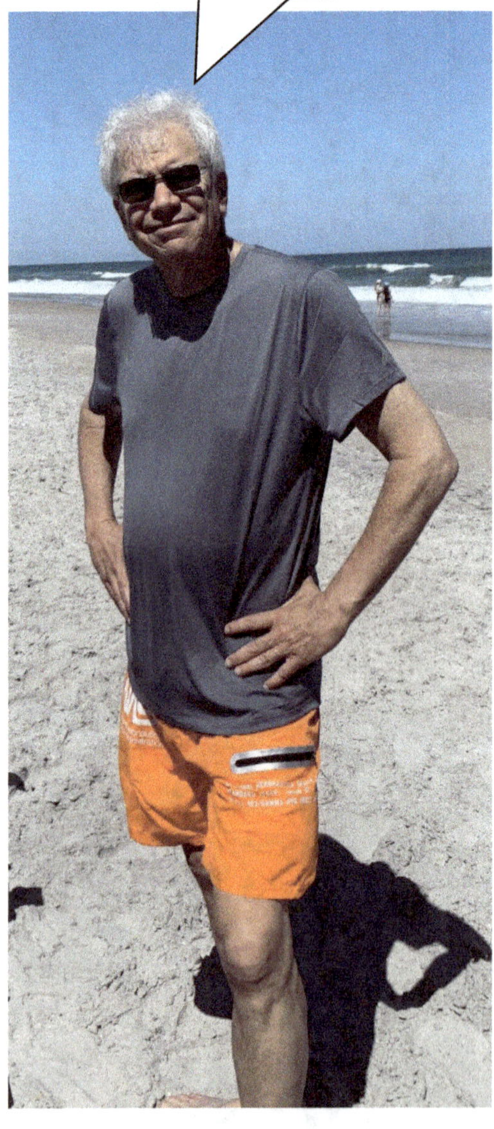
I hope you found this
book useful. Good luck!